Table Of Contents

Introduction

Testicular disease happens when cells in the gonad develop to frame a growth. This is intriguing. In excess of 90% of testicular tumors start in the microbe cells, which produce sperm. There are two kinds of microbe cell diseases (GCTs). Seminoma can develop gradually and answer to radiation and chemotherapy. Non-seminoma can develop all the more rapidly and can be less receptive to those medicines. There are a couple of kinds of non-seminomas: choriocarcinoma, embryonal carcinoma, teratoma and yolk sac growths.

There are additionally uncommon testicular malignant growths that don't shape in the microbe cells. Leydig cell cancers structure from the Leydig cells that produce testosterone. Sertoli cell cancers emerge from the Sertoli cells that help ordinary sperm development. Testicular growths can be made of more than one kind of cell.

The sort of testicular malignant growth cell found, side effects and different elements will assist with directing your treatment.

Chapter One

Testicular Cancer

Testicular malignant growth is disease that creates in the balls, a piece of the male regenerative framework. Side effects might remember a knot for the gonad or expanding or torment in the scrotum. Treatment might bring about barrenness.

Risk factors incorporate an undescended testis, family background of the illness, and past history of testicular disease. Over 95% are microorganism cell growths which are partitioned into seminomas and non-seminomas. Different sorts incorporate sex-rope stromal growths and lymphomas. Finding is regularly founded on an actual test, ultrasound, and blood tests. Careful expulsion of the gonad with assessment under a magnifying instrument is then finished to decide the sort.

Testicular disease is profoundly treatable and normally reparable.

Therapy choices might incorporate a medical procedure, radiation treatment, chemotherapy, or undeveloped cell transplantation. Indeed, even in cases in which malignant growth has spread broadly, chemotherapy offers a fix rate more prominent than 80%.

Around the world testicular disease impacted around 686,000 individuals in 2015. That year it brought about 9,400 passings up from 7,000 passings in 1990. Rates are lower in the creating than the created world. Beginning most ordinarily happens in guys 20 to 34 years of age, seldom before 15 years of age. The five-year endurance rate in the US is around 95%. Results are better when the illness stays limited.

Chapter Two

Signs and Symptoms

One of the principal indications of testicular malignant growth is in many cases an irregularity or expanding in the testicles. The U.S. Preventive Administrations Team (USPSTF) advises against routine evaluating for testicular malignant growth in asymptomatic juvenile and grown-ups including routine testicular self-tests. Nonetheless, the American Malignant growth Society proposes that a few men ought to inspect their gonads month to month, particularly on the off chance that they have a family background of disease, and the American Urological Affiliation suggests month to month testicular self-assessments for every single young fellow.

Side effects may likewise incorporate at least one of the accompanying:

- An irregularity in one testis which could conceivably be excruciating.
- Sharp torment or a dull throb in the lower mid-region or scrotum.
- An inclination frequently depicted as "weight" in the scrotum.
- Solidness of the gonad.
- Bosom broadening (gynecomastia) from hormonal impacts of β-hCG.
- Low back torment (lumbago) because of the malignant growth spreading to the lymph hubs along the back.

It isn't extremely normal for testicular malignant growth to spread to different organs, aside from the lungs. On the off chance that it has, nonetheless, the accompanying side effects might be available:

•Windedness (dyspnea), hack or hacking up blood (hemoptysis) from metastatic spread to the lungs.
•A protuberance in the neck because of metastases to the lymph hubs.

Testicular disease, cryptorchidism, hypospadias, and unfortunate semen quality spread the word about up the disorder as testicular dysgenesis condition.

14

Chapter Three

Causes

A significant gamble factor for the improvement of testis disease is cryptorchidism (undescended gonads). It is for the most part accepted that the presence of a growth adds to cryptorchidism;

when cryptorchidism happens related to a cancer then the cancer will in general be huge. Other gamble factors incorporate inguinal hernias, Klinefelter disorder, and mumps orchitis. Actual work is related with diminished risk and stationary way of life is related with expanded risk. Beginning stage of male qualities is related with expanded risk. These may reflect endogenous or ecological chemicals.

Higher paces of testicular disease in Western countries have been connected to the utilization of marijuana.

17

Chapter Four

Mechanisms

Most testicular microorganism cell cancers have an excessive number of chromosomes, and most frequently they are triploid to tetraploid. An isochromosome 12p (the short arm of chromosome 12 on the two sides of a similar centromere) is available in around 80% of the testicular diseases, and furthermore different malignant growths normally have additional material from this chromosome arm through different systems of genomic enhancement.

Chapter Five

Diagnosis

The main way testicular cancer is diagnosed is via a lump or mass inside a testis. More generally, if a young adult or adolescent has a single enlarged testicle, which may or may not be painful, this should give doctors reason to suspect testicular cancer.

Different circumstances may likewise have side effects like testicular disease:

•Epididymitis or epididymo-orchitis

•Hematocele

•Varicocele

•Orchitis

•Prostate diseases or aggravations (prostatitis), bladder contaminations or irritations (cystitis), or kidney (renal) contaminations (nephritis) or irritations which have spread to and caused expanding in the vessels of the balls or scrotum.

•Testicular twist or a hernia.

•Contamination, aggravation, retro-peritonitis, or different states of the lymph hubs or vessels close to the scrotum, balls, pubis, anorectal region, and crotch.

•Harmless growths or sores of the gonads

•Metastasis to the balls from another, essential cancer site(s).

The idea of any touched irregularity in the scrotum is many times assessed by scrotal ultrasound, which can decide precise area, size, and a few qualities of the bump, for example, cystic versus strong, uniform versus heterogeneous, pointedly encompassed or ineffectively characterized. The degree of the sickness is assessed by CT filters, which are utilized to find metastases.

The differential finding of testicular disease requires looking at the histology of tissue acquired from an inguinal orchiectomy - that is, careful extraction of the whole testis alongside connected structures (epididymis and spermatic rope). A biopsy ought not be performed, as it raises the gamble of spreading malignant growth cells into the scrotum.

Inguinal orchiectomy is the favored strategy since it brings down the gamble of malignant growth cells getting away. This is on the grounds that the lymphatic arrangement of the scrotum, through which white platelets (and, possibly, disease cells) stream in and out, connections to the lower limits, while that of the gonad connects to the rear of the stomach cavity (the retroperitoneum). A trans-scrotal biopsy or orchiectomy will possibly leave disease cells in the scrotum and make two courses for malignant growth cells to spread, while in an inguinal orchiectomy just the retroperitoneal course exists.

Blood tests are additionally used to distinguish and gauge growth markers (normally proteins present in the circulatory system) that are well defined for testicular disease. Alpha-fetoprotein, human chorionic gonadotropin (the "pregnancy chemical"), and LDH-1 are the regular cancer markers used to recognize testicular microorganism cell growths.

A pregnancy test might be utilized to recognize elevated degrees of chorionic gonadotropin; nonetheless, the primary indication of testicular disease is typically an effortless irregularity. Note that just around 25% of seminomas have raised chorionic gonadotropin, so a pregnancy test isn't extremely delicate for making out testicular disease.

Screening

The American Institute of Family Doctors advises against evaluating guys without side effects for testicular malignant growth.

Staging

After evacuation, the gonad is fixed with Bouin's answer since it better rations a few morphological subtleties like atomic compliance.

Then the testicular growth is organized by a pathologist as per the TNM Grouping of Dangerous Growths as distributed in the AJCC Disease Organizing Manual. Testicular malignant growth is classified as being in one of three phases (which have subclassifications). The size of the growth in the testis is unimportant to organizing. In expansive terms, testicular disease is organized as follows:

•Stage I: the disease stays restricted to the testis.
•Stage II: the disease includes the testis and metastasis to

retroperitoneal and additionally paraaortic lymph hubs (lymph hubs underneath the stomach).

•Stage III: the disease includes the testis and metastasis past the retroperitoneal and paraaortic lymph hubs. Stage 3 is additionally partitioned into non-massive stage 3 and cumbersome stage 3.

Additional data on the itemized organizing framework is accessible on the site of the American Disease Society.

Classification

Albeit testicular disease can be gotten from any cell type tracked down in the gonads, over 95% of testicular malignant growths are microbe cell cancers (GCTs). The vast majority of the leftover 5% are sex line gonadal stromal cancers got from Leydig cells or Sertoli cells. Right conclusion is important to guarantee the best and fitting treatment. Somewhat, this should be possible by means of blood tests for growth markers, however conclusive finding requires assessment of the histology of an example by a pathologist.

Most pathologists utilize the World Wellbeing Association grouping framework for testicular cancers:

•Microbe cell cancers
  °Antecedent sores
    -Microbe cell neoplasia in situ
    -Unclassified sort (carcinoma in situ)
    -Determined types

  °Cancers of one histologic sort (unadulterated structures)
    -Seminoma
    -Variation - Seminoma with syncytiotrophoblastic cells
    -Spermatocytic cancer

-Variation - spermatocytic cancer with sarcoma

-Embryonal carcinoma

-Yolk sac cancer

-Trophoblastic cancers

-Choriocarcinoma

-Variation - monophasic choriocarcinoma

-Placental site trophoblastic cancer

-Cystic trophoblastic cancer

Teratoma

-Variation - Dermoid growth

-Variation - Epidermoid growth

-Variation - Monodermal teratoma (Carcinoid), Crude neuroectodermal cancer (PNET), Nephroblastoma-like growth, others.

-Variation - Teratomic with substantial sort danger

°Cancers of more than one histologic sort (blended structures)
-Embryonal carcinoma and teratoma
-Teratoma and seminoma
-Choriocarcinoma and teratoma. Embryonal carcinoma
-Others

•Sex rope/Gonadal stromal cancers
°Leydig cell growth
°Sertoli cell growth
-Lipid rich variation
-Sclerosing variation

-Enormous cell calcifying variation

-Intratubular Sertoli cell neoplasia in Peutz-Jeghers disorder

°Granulosa cell growth
   -Grown-up type
   -Adolescent sort

°Thecoma fibroma bunch
   -Thecoma
   -Fibroma

°Sex line/gonadal stromal cancer - not entirely separated
°Sex line/gonadal stromal cancer - blended types

•Blended microorganism cell and sex line/gonadal stromal growths
  °Gonadoblastoma
  °Microorganism cell-sex line/gonadal stromal growth, unclassified

•Different cancers of the testis
  °Lymphomas
    -Essential testicular diffuse enormous B-cell lymphoma
    -Mantle cell lymphoma of the testicles
    -Extranodal minor zone B cell lymphoma of the testicles
    -Extranodal NK/Immune system microorganism lymphoma, nasal kind of the testicles

-Fringe Immune system microorganism lymphoma of the testicles

-Activin receptor-like kinase-1-negative anaplastic enormous cell lymphoma of the testicles

-Pediatric-type follicular lymphoma of the testicles

°Carcinoid

°Growths of ovarian epithelial sorts
-Serous growth of marginal threat
-Serous carcinoma
-Very much separated endometrioid growth
-Mucinous cystadenoma
-Mucinous cystadenocarcinoma

-Brenner growth

°Nephroblastoma

°Paraganglioma

•Haematopoietic growths
•Growths of gathering channels and rete
  °Adenoma
  °Carcinoma

•Growths of the paratesticular structures
  °Adenomatoid growth
  °Threatening and harmless mesothelioma

°Adenocarcinoma of the epididymis

°Papillary cystadenoma of the epididymis

°Melanotic neuroectodermal growth

°Desmoplastic little round cell growth

•Mesenchymal growths of the spermatic rope and testicular adnexae

°Lipoma

°Liposarcoma

°Rhabdomyosarcoma

°Forceful angiomyxoma

°Angiomyofibroblastoma-like growth (see Myxoma)

°Fibromatosis
°Fibroma
°Singular sinewy growth
°Others
•Auxiliary growths of the testis

Chapter Six

Treatment

The three fundamental kinds of therapy are a medical procedure, radiation treatment, and chemotherapy.

Medical procedure is performed by urologists; radiation treatment is directed by radiation oncologists; and chemotherapy is crafted by clinical oncologists. In many patients with testicular malignant growth, the illness is restored promptly with negligible long haul dismalness. While therapy achievement relies upon the stage, the typical endurance rate following five years is around 95%, and stage 1 malignant growth cases, whenever checked appropriately, have basically a 100 percent endurance rate.

Gonad evacuation

The underlying therapy for testicular malignant growth is a medical procedure to eliminate the impacted gonad (orchiectomy). While it could be conceivable, at times, to eliminate testicular disease growths from a testis while leaving the testis useful, this is never finished, as the impacted gonad ordinarily contains pre-malignant cells spread all through the whole gonad. In this way eliminating the growth alone without extra therapy significantly builds the gamble that another disease will frame in that gonad.

Since only one testis is regularly expected to keep up with richness, chemical creation, and other male capabilities, the impacted testis is quite often taken out totally in a technique called inguinal orchiectomy. (The gonad is never eliminated through the scrotum; a cut is made underneath the belt line in the inguinal region.) In the UK, the technique is known as an extreme orchidectomy.

Retroperitoneal lymph hub analyzation

On account of non-seminomas that seem, by all accounts, to be stage I, medical procedure might be finished on the retroperitoneal/paraaortic lymph hubs (in a different activity) to precisely decide if the disease is in stage I or stage II and to diminish the gamble that threatening testicular malignant growth cells that might have metastasized to lymph hubs in the lower midsection. This medical procedure is called retroperitoneal lymph hub analyzation (RPLND). Be that as it may, this methodology, while standard in many spots, particularly the US, is undesirable because of expenses and the elevated degree of mastery expected to carry out effective procedure. Sperm banking is regularly completed preceding the method (similarly as with chemotherapy), as there is a gamble that RPLND might harm the nerves engaged with discharge, making discharge happen inside into the bladder instead of remotely.

Numerous patients are rather picking reconnaissance, where no further a medical procedure is performed except if tests demonstrate that the malignant growth has returned. This approach keeps a high fix rate in light of the developing precision of observation procedures.

Adjuvant treatment

Since testicular malignant growths can spread, patients are typically offered adjuvant therapy - as chemotherapy or radiotherapy - to kill any harmful cells that might exist beyond the impacted gonad. The sort of adjuvant treatment relies generally upon the histology of the cancer (i.e., the size and state of its cells under the magnifying instrument) and the phase of movement at the hour of medical procedure (i.e., how far cells have 'got away' from the gonad, attacked the encompassing tissue, or spread to the remainder of the body). In the event that the malignant growth isn't especially exceptional, patients might be offered cautious observation by occasional CT sweeps and blood tests, instead of adjuvant treatment.

Before 1970, endurance rates from testicular disease were low. Starting from the presentation of adjuvant chemotherapy, predominantly platinum-based drugs like cisplatin and carboplatin, the standpoint has improved considerably. Albeit 7000 to 8000 new instances of testicular malignant growth happen in the US yearly, simply 400 men are supposed to pass on from the illness.

In the UK, a comparable pattern has arisen: since enhancements in treatment, endurance rates have increased quickly to fix paces of more than 95%.

Radiation treatment

Radiation might be utilized to treat stage II seminoma diseases, or as adjuvant (safeguard) treatment on account of stage I seminomas, to limit the probability that little, non-noticeable cancers exist and will spread (in the inguinal and para-aortic lymph hubs). Radiation is insufficient against and is thusly never utilized as an essential treatment for non-seminoma.

Chapter Seven

Chemotherapy

Non-seminoma

Chemotherapy is the standard therapy for non-seminoma when the malignant growth has spread to different pieces of the body (that is, stage 2B or 3). The standard chemotherapy convention is three, or once in a while four, rounds of

Bleomycin-Etoposide-Cisplatin (BEP). BEP as a first-line treatment was first revealed by Teacher Michael Peckham in 1983. The milestone preliminary distributed in 1987 which laid out BEP as the ideal treatment was led by Dr. Lawrence Einhorn at Indiana College. Another option, similarly powerful treatment includes the utilization of four patterns of Etoposide-Cisplatin (EP).

Lymph hub medical procedure may likewise be performed after chemotherapy to eliminate masses abandoned (stage 2B or further developed), especially in the instances of huge non-seminomas.

Seminoma

As an adjuvant therapy, utilization of chemotherapy as an option in contrast to radiation treatment in the therapy of seminoma is expanding, on the grounds that radiation treatment seems to have more critical long haul aftereffects (for instance, interior scarring, expanded dangers of auxiliary malignancies, and so on.). Two dosages, or sometimes a solitary portion of carboplatin, commonly conveyed three weeks separated, is ending up an effective adjuvant treatment, with repeat rates in similar reaches as those of radiotherapy. The idea of carboplatin as a solitary portion treatment was created by Tim Oliver, Teacher of Clinical Oncology at Barts and The London Institute of Medication and Dentistry. In any case, extremely long haul information on the viability of adjuvant carboplatin in this setting don't exist.

Since seminoma can repeat a very long time after the essential growth is eliminated, patients getting adjuvant chemotherapy ought to stay careful and not expect they are relieved 5 years after treatment.

Chapter Eight

<u>Prognosis</u>

Therapy of testicular malignant growth is one of the examples of overcoming adversity of present day medication, with supported reaction to treatment in over 90% of cases, paying little heed to arrange. In 2011 by and large fix paces of over 95% were accounted for, and 80% for metastatic sickness — the best reaction by any strong growth, with further developed endurance being credited basically to compelling chemotherapy. By 2013 more than 96% of the 2,300 men analyzed every year in the U.K. were considered relieved, an ascent by close to a third since the 1970s, the improvement credited considerably to the chemotherapy drug cisplatin. In the US, when the sickness is treated while it is as yet confined, over the vast majority of individuals endure 5 years.

Reconnaissance

For some patients with stage I malignant growth, adjuvant (deterrent) treatment following a medical procedure may not be proper and patients will go through observation all things considered. The structure this observation takes, for example the sort and recurrence of examinations and the length time it ought to proceed, will rely upon the kind of malignant growth (non-seminoma or seminoma), however the point is to stay away from superfluous therapies in the numerous patients who are restored by their medical procedure, and guarantee that any backslides with metastases (auxiliary tumors) are distinguished early and relieved. This approach guarantees that chemotherapy as well as radiotherapy is simply given to the patients that need it. The quantity of patients eventually relieved is a similar involving observation as post-employable "adjuvant" medicines, yet the patients must be ready to follow a drawn out series of visits and tests.

For both non-seminomas and seminomas, reconnaissance tests by and large incorporate actual assessment, blood tests for growth markers, chest x-beams and CT filtering. Be that as it may, the prerequisites of an observation program contrast as per the kind of sickness since, for seminoma patients, backslides can happen later, and blood tests are not as great at showing backslide.

CT examines are performed on the mid-region (and now and again the pelvis) and furthermore the chest in certain clinics. Chest x-beams are progressively liked for the lungs as they give adequate detail joined with a lower misleading positive rate and fundamentally more modest radiation portion than CT.

The recurrence of CT checks during reconnaissance ought to guarantee that backslides are distinguished at a beginning phase while limiting the radiation openness.

For patients treated for stage I non-seminoma, a randomized preliminary (Clinical Exploration Committee TE08)showed that, when joined with the standard observation tests depicted over, 2 CT checks at 3 and a year were comparable to 5 more than 2 years in recognizing backslide at a beginning phase.

For patients treated for stage I seminoma who pick observation as opposed to going through adjuvant treatment, there have been no randomized preliminaries to decide the ideal recurrence of sweeps and visits, and the timetables shift generally across the world, and inside individual nations. In the UK there is a continuous clinical preliminary called TRISST. This is evaluating how frequently outputs ought to happen and whether attractive reverberation imaging (X-ray) can be utilized rather than CT examines. X-ray is being examined on the grounds that it doesn't open the patient to radiation thus, assuming it is demonstrated to be as great at distinguishing backslides, it very well might be desirable over CT.

For further developed phases of testicular malignant growth, and for those cases where radiation treatment or chemotherapy was managed, the degree of checking (tests) after therapy will shift based on the conditions, however regularly ought to be finished for a considerable length of time in straightforward cases and for longer in those with higher dangers of backslide.

Richness

A man with one excess testis might keep up with rich. Notwithstanding, sperm banking might be fitting for men who actually plan to have youngsters, since richness might be unfavorably impacted by chemotherapy and additionally radiotherapy. A man who loses the two gonads will be barren after the strategy, however he might choose for bank suitable, disease free sperm preceding the methodology.

Chapter Nine

<u>Epidemiology</u>

Universally testicular disease brought about 8,300 passings in 2013 up from 7,000 passings in 1990. Testicular malignant growth has the most noteworthy predominance in the U.S. what's more, Europe, and is unprecedented in Asia and Africa. Overall occurrence has multiplied since the 1960s, with the most noteworthy paces of predominance in Scandinavia, Germany, and New Zealand.

Albeit testicular disease is generally normal among men matured 15-40 years, it has three pinnacles: outset through the age of four as teratomas and yolk sac cancers, ages 25-40 years as post-pubertal seminomas and non-seminomas, and from age 60 as spermatocytic growths.

Microbe cell growths of the testis are the most widely recognized disease in young fellows between the ages of 15 and 35 years.

USA

In the US, around 8,900 cases are analyzed a year. The gamble of testicular disease in white men is around 4-5 times the gamble in people of color, and multiple times that of Asian American men. The gamble of testicular malignant growth in Latinos and Native Americans is between that of white and Asian men. The reason for these distinctions is obscure.

The UK

In the UK, roughly 2,000 individuals are analyzed a year. Over a long period, the gamble is about 1 of every 200 (0.5%). It is the sixteenth most normal disease in men. It represents under 1% of malignant growth passings in men (around 60 men kicked the bucket in 2012).

Chapter Ten

Foods For Testicular Health

With such a lot of health data readily available nowadays, it's dazzling how frequently we disregard the most straightforward answer for better wellbeing: eating right. What's more, with regards to testicular wellbeing for men, there are a wide exhibit of explicit dietary decisions that are demonstrated to help gonad wellbeing.

Cancer prevention agent rich natural products and veggies

Testicular disease can influence men of all ages and is the most ordinarily analyzed kind of malignant growth in young fellows, particularly those ages 30 to 39. Much malignant growth research today focuses to oxidative pressure and irritation being contributing elements. Considering that the gonads normally have less oxygenated blood stream, they're prime possibility for oxidative pressure.

You can assist with lessening your possibilities creating testicular malignant growth by eating food sources high in cell reinforcements, like berries. Blueberries, blackberries and strawberries have for quite some time been hailed for their high nutrient substance and cancer prevention agent properties.

Concentrates on well defined for a scope of disease types, including colon malignant growth and bosom malignant growth, highlight an immediate connection to eating berries and lower malignant growth risk, and the equivalent goes for testicular disease. Other cell reinforcement rich food varieties incorporate carrots, red and yellow chime peppers, yams, tomatoes, natural grapes, pomegranates and cherries.

Artichokes

These astounding looking edibles sneak up suddenly, particularly for their size. Artichokes contain chlorogenic corrosive, which has been displayed to diminish the gamble for particular kinds of malignant growth, type 2 diabetes and coronary illness.

Note that not all artichoke dishes convey a similar cell reinforcement clout. Everything revolves around how you cook them. Bubbling artichokes raises their cancer prevention agent content by multiple times though steaming them raises the cell reinforcement level by multiple times. Sadly, broiling artichokes might diminish their cell reinforcement profile.

Garlic and onions

One more motivation to partake in these brilliantly impactful flavors, awful breath and all, is that garlic and onions have been displayed to diminish testicular oxidative pressure in mice, decreasing disease risk all the while.

Selenium

Selenium-rich food sources, for example, salmon, shrimp and sardines can assist with forestalling issues like prostate disease, male fruitfulness issues and testicular malignant growth. You can likewise build your selenium consumption the vegetarian way by eating a lot of Brazil nuts, seeds and green vegetables.

Vitamin B5

Different examinations have shown that vitamin B5 is valuable to cholesterol levels and the treatment of diabetes in men. One concentrate out of Japan — it was directed on rodents yet has suggestions for human guys — showed vitamin B5 further developed blood levels of testosterone, sperm motility and generally testicular capability. A few decent wellsprings of vitamin B5 incorporate corn, broccoli, sunflower seeds, mushrooms and avocados.

Zinc

As well as being a critical part of semen, zinc has been displayed to help safeguard against cadmium-initiated testicular harmfulness. Cadmium is a natural poison to which the gonads are especially delicate, and it can unleash ruin on your endocrine framework and regenerative capability. Eating food varieties high in zinc, for example, poultry, shellfish, red meat and pumpkin seeds might assist with moderating the risks.

The key to solid balls is essentially as close as your neighborhood grocery store racks. Our dietary decisions consistently essentially influence our wellbeing over the long haul, and staying away from terrible healthful propensities is many times similarly as simple as beginning great ones.